Caregiver's
POETIC JOURNAL

Caregiver's Poetic Journal: Begin Healing from Grief and Loss Through Journaling
Copyright © 2024 Sandra Mohsan. All rights reserved.

All rights reserved. No part of this book shall be reproduced, stored in a retrieval system, or transmitted by any means; electronic, mechanical, photocopying, recording or otherwise, without written permission from the publisher, except for providing a direct quote and providing reference.

Please email Sandra@SandraMohsan.com for bulk discounts.

ISBN:
979-8-9918653-0-2   Paperback
979-8-9918653-1-9   Hardcover
979-8-9918653-2-6   Ebook

Editing: Robin Steinweg • RobinSteinweg.wixsite.com/my-site-1 | RobinSteinweg.com

Design: Bookable Media • BookableMedia.com

Images: Adobe Stock, Sandra Mohsan

Illustration: Sandra Marie Mohsan, CRN, BSN, PHN, TNP, Caritas Coach®, Pamela Dayon RN, BA, Caritas Coach®

Caregiver's
POETIC JOURNAL

Begin Healing from Grief and Loss

Through Journaling

SANDRA MOHSAN, CRN, BSN, PHN, TNP, CARITAS COACH®

Your Gift from Sandra

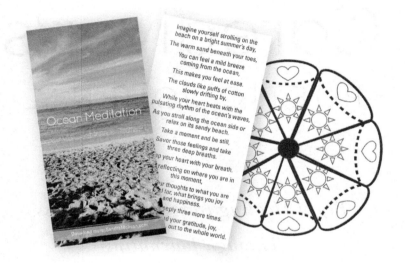

Thank you for your support and purchase of this book.
Please access your free gift from Sandra at the link below.

A meditation card you can download.
A mandala to explore your artistic talents.

SandraMohsan.com/gift

COMPASSIONATE REFLECTIONS

Caregiver's Poetic Journal takes readers on a lovely poetic journey into the inner recesses of your heart and its unfolding process along the way. An enlightening and inspiriting adventure into life itself with all its moods and moments.

Sandra's inspired creative expressions reflect common human bonds of loss and joy.

Jean Watson, PhD, RN, AHN-BC, FAAN, LL (AAN)
Founder, Director, Watson Caring Science Institute

As I read this book I felt moved by Sandra's exploring, loving, and transforming spirit. The engaging way she took care of her husband and accepted that lovingkindness for herself was profound. She writes from an authentic healing heart. I felt her beautiful energy jump off the page and land on my heart!

It was an honor to read her journey and story. I thoroughly enjoyed it and recommend it to anyone and everyone.

Marcy B. Newman, DACM, RN, MPH, Caritas Coach®,
Registered Nurse, Acupuncturist, iRestYoga Nidra,
Certified Teacher and RYT Certified Yoga Instructor

Sandra Mohsan's *Caregiver's Poetic Journal* is a beautifully moving experience of a nurse's personal journey of healing through profound loss, and of listening to and documenting her heart's voice with honesty and creativity.

Her words give us courage, and her humor lifts our spirits. In the face of the loss of her soulmate of forty years, she stays true to herself, her broken heart, and the reality of leaving her known professional work to become something and someone new.

As Sandra herself wrote in her *Caregiver's Poetic Journal*, "First for self, let the thoughts flow free, then they can be shared for all the world to see."

Anne Pera, RN, HN-BC, BSN, PHN, Reiki Master Teacher

The loss of a life partner is a journey into the raw depths of what it means to walk in the fullness of this human experience. It is a place where joys of the heart and unimaginable sorrows dance together. It is a reminder of how this life tugs us in every direction, removing all that we rely on, only to ask us to find our way through the wild mysteries of grief. To brave this journey is an invitation into awakening to that place where the heart opens so wide there is nothing left but love. Love that artists, poets, and spiritual teachers try in so many ways to point us to.

This is not a path for the faint of heart. It takes tremendous courage to enter the turbulence of transformation. By tending to her grief and sharing her authentic exploration of love and loss, Sandra offers a ray of hope. For some, a roadmap— toward understanding that the heart can break all the way open to the timeless, unbreakable place where love is found to be limitless.

Kathy Douglas, RN, MPH, CEO
The Nursing Way

In Sandy Mohsan's *Caregiver's Poetic Journal*
we journey through love, loss, and rebirth.
Her words are like a soothing balm, a warm
lantern, guiding us through the circle of life on Earth.

Her poetry carries the weight of sorrow and grief
yet dances in lightness and deep joy
with gratitude, forgiveness, and love to employ
navigating through life's moments brief.

Sandy's words inspire, uplift, and heal
her open heart a beacon in the dark
showing us a new perspective, a new zeal
a vision of life that leaves a lasting mark.

Janette V. Moreno, DNP, RN, NEA-BC, NPD-BC, Caritas Coach®,
Role-Driven Practice Coach, ANCC PTAP Appraiser, Executive Director, OIAPP

Sandra Mohsan has shared with her readers a poetic and insightful look into the caregiver and care receiver's relationship. She shares the struggle and the joy of capturing moments to refresh her spirit.

Readers will be inspired by Sandy's commitment to her husband, and her ability to find beauty and meaning in the journey.

Christine Blanke, RN, MS, CPH

COMPASSIONATE REFLECTIONS

Caregiver's Poetic Journal by Sandra Mohsan is a deeply moving and intimate portrayal of a caregiver's emotional journey through loss and grief. Sandra's heartfelt poetry reflects her experiences coping with significant life changes. Her words provide solace and insight into the complex emotions that accompany such profound loss.

For those who have experienced the passing of a loved one, Sandra's poetry can serve as a powerful tool for connection, empathy, and understanding. The act of writing poetry as a form of self-care is a deeply personal and therapeutic process, one that encourages us to honor our emotions and find healing through creative expression. *Caregiver's Poetic Journal* offers a poignant reminder to embrace our inner voice and allow poetry to be a source of comfort and healing as we navigate the challenges of illness and loss.

Grissel Hernandez, PhD, MPH, RN, HNB-BC, NPD-BC, SGAHN, Caritas Coach®, Watson Caring Science Postdoctoral Scholar, Executive Director, Professional Development, Education & Magnet Program, Center for Education & Professional Development, Stanford Health Care

When I had the joy years ago of sharing Dr. Jean Watson's Caring Science to nurses at the medical center where Sandra (Sandy) Mohsan served, she was one of those who lit up like a Christmas tree. Her face glowed with smiles because she'd found support in her life journey. Sandy grabbed it and went full force ahead.

Sandy's path quickly expanded to teaching others about Caring Science. She found that art and writing reached her heart the most. Caring Science pushed her more into the beautiful depths of her heart, especially by writing poems and journaling the pathway that she and her beloved husband were traveling.

Sandy has reached worldwide to touch other nurses with caring, communitas* and support: to care, to love, and to grieve together as we travel this life.

Pamela Dayon RN, BA, Caritas Coach®

Communitas carries several meanings, one of which is a *feeling of community*.

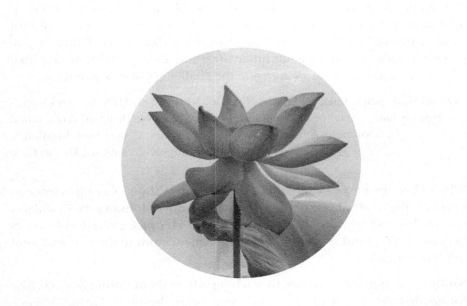

DEDICATION

This journal is dedicated to my husband, Muhammad Hamid Mohsan who passed away December 30, 2023, after battling metastatic mesothelioma for over eleven years. We were grateful for every treatment which helped prolong his life so we could be together. I will miss him, for we were soulmates for over forty years.

During his last few months of life, I struggled to maintain a job from home and care for him. Our family helped by cooking meals, escorting him to his treatments, making him comfortable, keeping us entertained, and allowing me time to rest. Eventually his health declined, and he required more assistance, so I retired early to be with him. This was one of the most difficult decisions I ever made.

I have shared our last days together in this journal. My friend, mentor, and colleague, Mary Rockwood Lane, inspired me to begin journaling as I attended her course, The Art of Nursing, The Healing Power of Artistic Expression. My journal entries usually were created as I sat in my sacred space every morning before starting the day. It was a time to reflect and gather my thoughts, which eventually blossomed into poetic form. The last poem in "Part I: Caregiver's Poetic Journey" brought an Ah-ha! moment, highlighting the importance of communication. The latter part of my journal was created as I attended Mary's course again. I was so blessed to have this experience, for I was given permission to express my grief and honor my sorrow through artistic expression: poetic journaling.

It was important to share my work with others going through loss and grief by demonstrating how journaling and using artistic talents can release one's innermost feelings, which then aids in the healing process of a broken heart.

It is also my hope for you, as you share my journal with me, that this becomes your beacon of light into how Caring Science/mindful practice, meditation, self-care, and unification with others will provide you with healing, solace, peace of mind, and equanimity as you, too, progress through your life's journey—a journey where you may embrace grief and loss.

CONTENTS

Compassionate Reflections v
Dedication ix
Foreword xv
Amazing Journey.. xix
My Hope for You xxi
Passing of Time xxii
Artistic Expression Validates the Nurse's Gifts, Talents,
and Wonderment xxiii
The Pain of Loss... xxiv

Part One: Caregiver's Poetic Journey 1

    September 30 Art and Play 2
    October 1   Love and Care 4
    October 2   Hope Sustaining.. 6
    October 3   Sign of the Times 8
    October 4   In the Darkness 10
    October 5   Healthcare Dance 12
    October 6   Self-care.. 14
    October 7   Love and Support....................................... 16
    October 8   Facing the World 18
    October 9   Let There be Light...................................... 20
    October 10   I am in Heaven 22
    October 11   The Time That is Mine 24
    October 12   Quantum Leap 26
    October 13   "Aye Calypso" 28
    October 14   Micro-Moments 30
    October 15   Faith and Lovingkindness 32
    October 16   Reflection 34

October 19	Negative and the Positive	36
October 20	The Closing of a Chapter	38
October 21	Retirement Day	40
October 22	When Will My Ship Sail?	42
October 23	Lead Me in the Right Direction	44
October 24	Seeking Counsel	46
October 25	Nerves are Tested	48
October 26	Patience	50
October 27	Missing Entry	52
October 28	Season Changing	54
October 29	Losing Control but Staying Strong by Practicing Lovingkindness	56
October 30	Fight the Pain	58
November 1	Respect	60
November 2	Exhaustion	62
November 3	Take a Deep Breath to Breathe in a New Day	64
November 4	Nap Time	66
November 7	A Thankful Reflection	68
November 9	Time is Not Mine	70
Nov. 10-22	Missing Entries	72
November 23	Returning	74
November 24	Thanksgiving Surprise	76
November 25	Blessings	78
November 26	Spread Lovingkindness Through My Writings and Poetry	80
November 27	Gratitude Through Music	82
November 28	Exhausting Day of Challenges	84
November 29	Dream on, You Say	86
November 30	Wintertime	88
December 1	The Importance of Communication	90
Caregiver's Poetic Journey: Loss of a Great Person		93

Part Two: Light in the Universe **97**

February 26	A Day of Firsts	98
February 27	Words are Left Behind	100
February 28	Honoring the Nurses	102
February 29	What a State I am in	104
March 1	A Bigger Bond Has Been Made	106
March 2	Grateful For Endless Treasures	108
March 3-4	A Cultural Connection	110
March 5	A New Adventure in Creativity	112
March 6	Forgiveness	114
March 7	Wishing You Were with Me	116
March 8	The Bread of Life	118
March 9	Intimate Moments	120
March 10	Happy Heavenly Birthday	122
March 11	My Work is Dedicated to You	124
March 12	Writer's Block	126
March 13	When We First Met	128
March 14	On a Do-Nothing Day	130
March 15	On a Do-Something Day	132
March 16	Reminiscing With a Friend	134
March 17	Miracle World	136
March 18	Need to Remember to Center Myself	138
March 19	Commemorating You	140
March 20	The Road is Not a Road; it is a Journey	142
March 21	The Scarf Dance	144
March 22	If Our Sacred Places Could Tell a Story	146
March 23	Ocean Meditation	148
March 24	Embrace Each Moment	150
March 25	Nurturing My Singing Voice	152
March 26	Place of Honor	154
March 27	A Poetic Verse from Me to You	156

March 28	Faced with Another First Without You	158
March 29	The Greatest Gift	160
March 30	My World of Artistic Expression	162
March 31	Happy Easter	164
April 1	Another First	166
April 2	A Chill Down My Spine	168
April 3	A Strawberry Éclair if You Dare	170
April 4	Poetry and Affirmation	172
April 5	Grateful for Tomorrow	174
April 6	Release of Tears, Self-Healing	176
April 7	Caritas Touch, so Divine	178
April 8	This Time I am not Late	180
April 7	Use the Fine China My Dear	182
April 10	Missing in Action	184
April 11	Eid Mubarak to You in the Heavens Above	186
April 12	So Many Things That You Used to Do	188
April 13	Late But Not Forgotten	190
April 14	Another Day of First: Taxes	192
April 15	Seven Sutras: Which one Sings to Me	194
April 15	The Image That I See	196
April 16	An Imposing Loss	198
April 19	Closure	200

About the Author	203
Resources	205
Thank you	206

FOREWORD

Caregiver's Poetic Journal takes us on a journey of love, loss, and rebirth as Sandra Mohsan shares her most precious moments in the form of poetic reflections that illustrate the circle of life and death as she cares for her husband of forty years, Muhammad.

Her reflections remind us of what we will all face and how the grace, beauty and strength of the human spirit when guided by love and care can help us through these times.

Sandy's poetry moves us with lightness, joy, loss, and deep sadness. Caring Science themes and practices are interwoven throughout her journey, along with reflections of caring as a registered nurse and wife during COVID, isolation, severe illness, death, her retirement, and the loss of her dear husband. She shares her many firsts and lasts and finds her sacred place as she deepens and grows toward inner peace. She keeps an open and loving heart filled with gratitude, acceptance, and love.

Even while her heart breaks, Sandy inspires and uplifts us to find a new perspective and vision of life.

Jan Anderson, EdD, RN, AHN-BC, Caritas Coach®

FOREWORD

Sandra Mohsan's warm smile first drew me in when we met in 2016 at The International Caritas Consortium hosted by Stanford Health Care in San Mateo, California. After her presentation she gave each of us a beautiful hand-painted rock which she distributed out of a basket lined with blue and white gingham. I was mesmerized.

She shared with me that her work entailed being the first point of contact for patients and families. "How wise," I thought, "that Kaiser Permanente Health has this kind soul to be the first encounter in what can otherwise be a frightening and daunting place, especially in a health crisis."

Throughout the years we've maintained a friendship, and I have watched her with great enthusiasm develop her wondrous artwork, and later, her profoundly moving, joyful, painful, real, and honest poetry.

How can we communicate when words are not available? How can we express our pain, our joy, or our sadness if not through such mediums as music, art, and storytelling? How can we understand a family member or a patient when speaking ceases to express what's really going on, or language is indecipherable?

As nurses, using my mother—Jean Watson's—10 Caritas Processes®, Process # 1 is about caring for self. Sandra is a perfect example of this process as she takes us with her on her own journey of grief, loss, joy, and celebration. Sandra has managed to reclaim her inner child artist, just as Picasso reminds us: "Every child is an artist. The problem is how to remain an artist once we grow up."

I celebrate Sandra's creations and am honored to be asked to write the foreword to her book. I know you will enjoy and benefit from it.

Julie Watson, BFA, MA, FRSA, Caritas Coach® Executive Director Watson Caring Science Institute Managing Editor, Lotus Library, Honorary Member, Sigma Theta Tau International, Honor Society of Nursing, Awarded "The Top 50 Women Leaders of Miami for 2023"—Article in *Fortune Business Magazine*

AMAZING JOURNEY

Where do I begin to share my amazing journey of enlightenment, peace, tranquility, equanimity, and healing? About seven years ago I was introduced to Jean Watson's Caring Science and Lovingkindness. My coworker, Caritas Coach®, and beloved friend Pamela Dayon introduced me to Jean's theory and presented me with one of Jean's CDs, "Caritas Meditation," which I listened to every day. My friend encouraged me to accompany her to my first Caritas Consortium, where I met Doctor Jean Watson.

The next adventure was to bring/bridge the knowledge and energy from that gathering to my work environment. Together we created posters illustrating Jean Watson's Theory and 10 Caritas Processes®, made breakout exercises available to nurses, which included a heart-centering moment and meditation cards, and we created a meditation tape and a Caring Science Introductory PowerPoint Presentation.

My colleague and beloved friend then encouraged and mentored me through the Caritas Coach® Program, which opened my eyes to a whole new world of lovingkindness and transpersonal caring. The program continued to make me aware of the awesomeness of Jean's theory and Caritas Processes. I was being/becoming and developing my Caritas-literate skills and strengthening my knowings, my inner spirit and creativity, and making transpersonal, lasting and caring connections with my new colleagues.

During the program I witnessed an abundance of energy and expansion of creativity through writing, poetry, dance, music, and artwork. I wanted to share my new knowledge of what it felt like to "be/being/becoming" Caritas literate to my colleagues and co-workers. Our mission was to educate and enlighten our professional colleagues and open their hearts to the lovingkindness of Caring Science.

Developing Caritas Literacy through education has the potential to transform the culture and atmosphere of not only our work environment, but that of the institution—by enhancing job satisfaction, providing a sense of being/becoming/belonging to a group of professional health care providers who exemplify high quality performance and community service.

As Jean Watson has said, Caring Science can be a primary influence on nursing education, care of patients, administrative practices and even research.

Today I will embark on a new journey of firsts: firsts without my soulmate of forty-two years, where the practice of self-care, self-reflection, and healing will be my primary goal. Along this journey I hope to enlighten others with what I have experienced and learned.

MY HOPE FOR YOU

My hope for you is that you will find a way to begin healing from your grief and loss, embrace your innermost thoughts and feelings, and record those precious moments through journaling.

During the last few months of taking care of my husband Muhammad, I attended a course with Mary Rockwood Lane called The Art of Nursing. She encouraged us to keep a journal. As I wrote, my thoughts were expressed in poetic form. Our group was then invited to return to her next session, and my second journal was created. This time the course was after Muhammad's passing. The journal again presented itself poetically. I combined them to create my book about this adventure and titled it *Caregiver's Poetic Journal.*

I felt it was important to share my work with others who are going through grief and loss because through journaling and using artistic expression, we can release our inner thoughts and feelings. This will help in the healing process.

1. Take time in your day to open this journal in a quiet place.
2. On the left will be my journal entry.
3. The right side is designed for you to share your reflections: a place to record your precious moments—perhaps a sketch, a poem, or a photo.
4. Interspersed throughout the book, you'll find Questions for Reflection to guide you in releasing your thoughts and feelings.
5. Visit SandraMohsan.com and share your story to receive a gift for taking time to read about my journey.

Passing of Time

When a loved one is terminally ill, we anticipate their passing and begin a journey of acceptance. Their life's timeline has been laid out before them. We may contemplate our own mortality because of this. Sometimes our loved one is taken from us abruptly, leaving us without time to prepare. Whether the process is gradual or sudden, the loss feels final, and we need help to process it all. We can watch for rays of hope to come to us—perhaps family or friends showing up in unexpected ways, or in the case of illness, a treatment that allows you a little more time together. Time will never erase your loved one, but it can bring a measure of healing to the heart.

Artistic Expression Validates the Nurse's Gifts, Talents, and Wonderment

Have you ever stopped to feel
What it is inside that makes you real?

How do you express what you have inside
Especially after a difficult day, when you want to cry?

Or if your day has brought you great gladness
How do you celebrate this happiness?

How do you go about your day?
When in a demanding situation, what makes you stay?

What keeps you motivated in these times?
What keeps you coming back to save more lives?

What artistic gifts, talents, wonderments have been bestowed?
How has this rejuvenated you? To what do you hold?

To begin your exploration, reach deep inside your mind to start
Artistic expression validates the gifts, talents, and wonderment that resonate from the heart.

The Pain of Loss

The pain of loss: wretched, my soul
Loss is so painful, you know.

My birthday is today, and you were not here
I hold back the tears.

They will flow, but not now
For the day has just begun—so much to do, places to be.

I know you don't want me to cry
But it's so hard to say goodbye.

The music I listen to opens my heart and soul
Embracing my thoughts about you makes me feel not alone—
but complete, whole.

As I go about this earthly world, this earthly world without you
Remember to smile on me and I will smile with you.

PART ONE

Caregiver's Poetic Journey

Art and Play
September 30

Look what I got today
Now I'm ready to create and play.

Prior to my own gift-surprise
I gathered all my art supplies

From our grandson's room, and there was plenty
I was in heaven and said these were many,

Many supplies to explore, create
For the sky would be the limit on what I could make.

I placed my supplies on the kitchen table
Heartfelt, ready to craft as I please

But to my surprise an emergency arose
Sometimes that happens, and nobody knows

How your best laid-out plans take you down a different path and
You discover your crafting supplies fall into someone else's hands.

My grandson thought I gathered them for him
They were hidden in his room, and he had forgotten about them.

To my surprise when I returned from my hospital stay
The table was empty and the art supplies had gone astray.

After finding out where they mysteriously went
I was overjoyed; then to Amazon we went.

My daughter at the helm, we found a package of colorful tools galore
And to my surprise early this morning it was outside my door.

Thank you, Sophia

Personal Reflection

Love and Care
October 1

The day has just begun
Or did the day before and today blur into one?

Hard to tell, for my mind is a whirl
Lack of sleep makes me a forgetful girl.

Time to get up and see what you need
Did you sleep at all, and are you comfortable?

Rough night, I see, and not pain free
Time for intervention—and that would be me.

Pain meds and a little adjustment here and there
The pain is a little less, and easier to bear.

Morning meds given early to smooth the routine
And then it is off to take care of me.

Now the bed is made, I'm dressed, hair in place, ready to go
We mustn't forget breakfast and the cat, you know.

Morning routine is on its way
Remember not to forget to journal in my poetic way.

Our cat Simba and I are in our sacred place
Spending a few minutes before plunging into our daily race.

As a caregiver now, you see
I will also need you to take care of me.

I'll need time to regenerate, power up my pack
I'll be fully functional. What do you think of that?

I love you so as we journey together
Remembering when we vowed, we'd be together forever.

Close your eyes and take a rest
And I'll pick up the pieces and do my best

To comfort you, take care of the cat
And not forget myself.

Personal Reflection

Hope Sustaining
October 2

Up early, as you can see
Making sure you're okay as you say good morning to me.

Too dark to see our sacred space
But it's this moment in time we need to begin to pace—

Pace out the morning and today's events
Nothing like being prepared for what's next.

No worry if you have a lack of sleep
For what sleep you had was very deep.

Naps are great to catch up
We will nap today, you and me.

This is a cool shift as caregiver, you know
For a four-hour breaktime nightly in this 24/7 show.

Now for breakfast as the crew is awake
Time to get up, offer the cat his potty break.

Rejuvenated and reenergized, breakfast I will make
Hope it turns out and I don't make a mistake.

Up from my sacred space
Time to take hold before running the daily race

But remember, it took these few minutes
To start my day first so I can take care of you.

Personal Reflection

Sign of the Times
October 3

My mind has been a whirl to see what this entry would be
Yesterday all day I considered writing about me.

Well, here goes, if you want to listen and sit down
I believe it'll tickle your funny bone; not make you frown.

Each morning when I wake
I pass the bathroom mirror, look in, yes that's me, no mistake.

As I comb and braid my long hair
The streak of white begins to appear.

This is the sign of my valor and achievements throughout the years
A sign of the times of happiness, joy, and tears.

Trimmed only once since COVID arrived
I have grown quite attached to it, a true symbol of life.

When I am done braiding, the white hair flows
regally in and out of the others.

I wonder how long I can get it to grow
I might stop when it reaches my toes.

All right, I'm ready for another day to begin
Time for breakfast; What creative adventures can I get in?

Personal Reflection

In the Darkness
OCTOBER 4

Am I still alive?

Up at 3 a.m.
Not sure where I am.

You needed assistance
I'm here as I rush to you from a distance.

Now you are all fluffed up and your concerns have been met
It's time for me to go back to bed.

But I'm awake, now that I can see
I'll stay up with the cat next to me.

I see the cat and he's gone back to sleep
I was hoping that would soon happen to me.

It's too dark to open the door to our sacred space
I will still journal in this place.

Not sure what this entry will entail as the morning hours tick by
With the effort to make it happen, I let out a sigh.

Spell check will be later, for it's hard to see
Time to go back to sleep, the cat and me.

Personal Reflection

Healthcare Dance
October 5

I did not end up in my sacred space this morning
I had breakfast with my honey.

The healthcare dance: what does it involve
Does it involve skipping down the halls?

Not at all, indeed
Just take a lesson from me.

It involves movement and coordination
To provide care without provocation.

It starts out with a good night's sleep
And if you get it, it's so sweet.

Morning hellos are first on the list
And then the morning medications you don't want to miss.

Requests are met, and then downstairs to make the first meal of the day
It's important to choreograph in a certain way

The meal is delivered hot and steamy
And we can sit together, you and me.

This is a dance that's learned by experience
Getting it right might seem serious

Don't worry, it will come with time
The perfection of the Healthcare Dance will be yours and mine.

You discover what works and what keeps breakfast warm
A Pakistani "Hot Pot" becomes the norm.

A hot towel is provided by the water from the carafe
Sometimes the water is too hot.

With patience it will cool
And breakfast will be ready for you.

We sit down and enjoy a meal
Discussing the dance for the day makes it more real

Let's sit and watch our favorite show
Then we can get ready to go

On to the next phase of the Healthcare Dance
One that's been perfected, one that will last.

Questions for Reflection

Have you had time to sit with the one you are caring for and hold their hand? Just sit quietly, intentionally aware. What did you experience?

Self-care
October 6

Today is journal day number seven
Another day up early, too dark even to see the heavens.

To my surprise
I'm sitting in my sacred space and opening my eyes.

Eyes and ears open at 6 a.m.
Wondering why I'm up so early and who I am

I'm not alone
When I open the patio door to the world, cars on the freeway sound
like waves of the sea.

We don't live close to the freeway
But the noise echoes and comes our way.

Many people up and moving around
As for me, I'd rather be in bed not making a sound.

Here I am in all my glory
Trying to jumpstart my morning.

I better get some coffee in me fast
I am not going to last.

Coffee in me, then ready to go
Perhaps conquer another assignment? Too early to know.

It's enough for now, time to take care of me.

Personal Reflection

Love and Support
October 7

I believe I must journal in my head
But you ask me to write down things instead.

The first time my thoughts begin to appear
It's in front of the bathroom mirror, I fear.

I start by admiring my pride
In the ribbon of courage that doesn't always hide.

Yes, it's the white streak, that band of white hair
That wraps strikingly around my braid.

Today is different as you can see
My hair is all over, no braid for me.

The night was rough; the night was bad
I stood watch with whatever I had.

I sit by your bedside and pass my time
Listening to a conference.

I must have passed out—exhaustion of mine
For the class was done, and that was fine.

There will be time to repeat it, you know
I went back to watching your breaths coming slow.

You're comfortable now so I can leave and retire
To my bed for a brief time until you desire

Desire or need additional care
Up and semi-dressed, I am there.

The day goes on and the grandkids entertain
Efforts to lighten you reduce some strain.

The strain and the worry you keep inside
While we, the family, work on issues outside.

It takes a village to keep things together
And to realize what really matters.

I am handed a bowl of warm bread pudding to devour
You look at me like you think the pudding is sour.

One bite and you warm inside, and I see you smile
Joy and happiness, pain-free—but just for a while.

It's all that matters in this moment in time
When you're overcome with equanimity, peace, and everything is fine

Personal Reflection

Facing the World
October 8

Poem nine and all is fine
Up in time.

Sitting in our sacred space
Looking out at the world we face.

We witness a water show
As the sprinklers flow.

No birds or squirrels that I can see
So that is how it'll be.

For a little while as all wake
It won't be long before the morning takes place.

Grandkids wake, and morning brings
Another day when the birds begin to sing.

Personal Reflection

Let There be Light
October 9

We're up early, and it's too dark to see
The birds, the squirrels, or even the trees.

The sound of traffic bustles overhead
It makes me think I'd rather be in bed.

Instead, I'll take advantage of it all
To turn on the lights; light up the halls.

Today is a big day for you and me
The day we go for your MRI.

You're afraid and up all night
Just going for the procedure causes you fright.

It'll be done and over with soon
Then our normal day can resume.

It's a holiday, but I hope some places are open for business
I have tasks that need to be tackled—within limits.

The reason I say within limits is my lack of sleep
A promise of the day will be a nap which I plan to keep.

I'm finally done with twenty-five units of continuing education
The information and excitement just swimming in my head.

Now time to focus on the next forty units
Time to relax, kick back, and enjoy.

The wonderment and creativity Mary Rockwood Lane brings
I am there, I'm open, I'm excited, I am everything!

Personal Reflection

I am in Heaven
OCTOBER 10

Entry eleven
I am in heaven

I just finished the draft of my short new story
About a yellow-and-black-striped fish in all her glory.

You see, she would not smile; her teeth were crooked and crowded
She spent most of her day away from other fish, and pouted.

She wouldn't smile, which gave her parents a fright
They wanted to help her to make things right.

Off to the orthodontist in Bodega Bay
To start her treatment that day.

She maintained fabulous self-care
Of her teeth and brace-wear

After some time, the braces were removed
And she smiled so bright and bodacious at the sun and the moon.

That was one happy fish, and so am I, since I was able to sleep last night.

Personal Reflection

The Time That is Mine
October 11

I got my days straight on my journal entry
Now I can begin to write freely.

Up early again today
Sun is not up yet and says no way.

Simba the Cat is with me
Starting his day but not very cuddly.

I cannot imagine my brain working at this time
Being motivated does happen, so I begin to rhyme.

Unbelievably this goes on all day
In my head I rehearse my next journal entry—what I'm going to say.

Poetic verses pop in and out
Some float away, others are written and scattered about.

The real time is here, where I can say what's on my mind
The time in my sacred space, the time that is mine.

Questions for Reflection

What creative activity have you done together today?
Have you taken time to share a story or listen to a song together?

Quantum Leap
October 12

Up early, as you see
For a very dark morning at six thirty.

Simba is on his tower watching his screen-time TV
While I'm writing away and feeling happy.

Why should I be happy so early, you ask
I'm up early to complete some tasks.

Paperwork, paperwork, paperwork and more
Will be the topic for what seems evermore.

But—and but, I say
There is light at the end of the tunnel. There must be a way

To make the next transition of my life appear
Smooth, effortless, and without fear,

I've decided to take a quantum leap and retire
Retire—and jump from the frying pan into the fire.

I must retire early; I don't know if I can be a 24/7 caregiver
And work forty hours a week; just thinking about it makes me shiver.

How will this time off work be covered? It isn't clear
How my benefits can be stretched out so I can care for you, dear.

I made the decision; the quantum leap that's key
To me being there for you and remain fully me.

Now I must run the pace of a jackrabbit
To contact my manager, Human Resources, and Retirement.

There's Social Security and Medicare
Call any of these places, if you dare.

You can wait on the phone for four hours or more
For them to tell you they can't help, give another phone number,
or shut the door.

It will be a couple of weeks of a rough road
A month or two till I'm paid, I'm told.

Now it's off to my savings to dive right in
To have this behind me; let the beauty and wonderment
of retirement begin.

Personal Reflection

"Aye Calypso"
October 13

Late, almost forgot to create an entry

"Aye Calypso" and Under the Sea"
What was I thinking to make me forget about me?

What a day I had; it started early
A lot better than yesterday, and did I go!

Started a hard copy of my journal so far
A binder so bright you can see it from afar.

I finished the videos and caught up with the class
I fell asleep this evening as the night hours passed.

Up once again to give the last evening med
Then back to bed as I crawl in to rest my head.

Personal Reflection

Micro-Moments
October 14

Micro-moments and micro gestures of kindness mean so much to me
Not only to give them, but to receive.

This morning, we worked on the menu and activity list
There was one additional gesture—a minor shift

From the usual routine to make the day go right
One we can agree on without a fight.

Where to position the lavender-scented trash basket so
There's less trash for me to pick up?

It's positioned close to the head of the bed on the floor
To hit it directly we need to calculate velocity and more!

Basket now positioned below your hand
When in bed we can figure out where it will land.

Wadding up more than one tissue might do the trick
Then you see the problem of trash on the floor will be licked.

Open minded after finally a good night's sleep
Let's see what other challenges we can meet,

Keeping in mind that micro-moments and micro gestures
of kindness to me
Mean so much—not only to give but receive.

Personal Reflection

Faith and Lovingkindness
October 15

Dark again this morning as we wake
Looks more like winter is approaching, no mistake.

Not too cold as I sip my coffee with delight
Feeling comfortable in a warm sweater, exactly right.

Just had an idea I might be able to catch my favorite morning show
Also open my messages before I begin to go—

Go, or dive into the day
Not sure if it will be all business or if I'll have some time to play.

I finally caught up and completed my class
Even caught up with some sleep as the night hours passed.

New energy, rejuvenated now
Many things to do, but not sure how

Can there be so many things that must be accomplished in a day
It will take time to see how this new journey will play.

I see so many friends who have passed into retirement limelight
For me, it causes fright.

I dreamt of having energy to clean up and de-junk my place
I'm not sure I can keep up that pace.

The pace or place where the mind thinks it should be
Where the body believes sleep is the reality.

I guess all those years of get-up and go
Eating quickly or not at all lets me know

Why it was said that I needed to take things slow
Take those deep breaths before I go—

Go to the room or call to assist the next patient I'd see
Now, it is time to take a deep breath before taking care of me.

I'm not sure about this new journey, but with faith and lovingkindness
the ride will be an interesting one, one where I won't be alone.

I'll have family, friends, and Simba. It's a brand-new world out there,
and here I come.

Personal Reflection

Reflection
OCTOBER 16

Up early today to write what I reflect on
Not too sure what the day will bring.

Personal Reflection

Negative and the Positive
October 19

I'm not sure this entry will be made as a poetic verse
I'm very tired, but things could be worse

I did get some sleep
I'll take a deep breath of relief.

It's sad that I was too busy to write
In my journal with the morning light

I thought I'd take it as my project in class when I go
Instead, I was so upset the last few mornings, I have nothing to show.

I've been working on my emergency retirement for days
Paperwork surrounding my table—I'm in a daze.

I wake up early; about 5 a.m.
When my normal routine would be to get started around ten.

At this magical hour there's not much to see
A couple of homes lit like Christmas trees.

Hmm, did I hear the bustling of cars this morning
Or did I just now notice it? My brain has been soaring.

Soaring since the countdown for the last day will be here
When the final chapter in my profession draws near.

But don't fret
It's not over yet

When the sea of paperwork settles down, I'll be free
To start my new professional journey.

Writing, teaching, and researching are what I have in mind.

Personal Reflection

The Closing of a Chapter
October 20

So many ideas swirling in my head
Ready to write so they stay there instead.

Breakfast done, laundry started, and coffee consumed
Sitting quietly at the table and then very soon

The birds should start chirping and the squirrel scamper by
This is the best part of the day, I cannot lie.

Tomorrow will be exciting too, but with a twist to see
It will be a big day for me.

I hope to open my company computer once more,
Close out my programs and delete what's been stored.

I hope to donate my knowledge and projects stored inside
So someone can continue my work with pride.

Many ideas and projects not complete
But someone to carry on, so I don't feel defeat.

I started to spread the Caritas word
Many years ago, and thought I was not heard

It was like a whisper that's now known three call-centers wide
I wear that accomplishment with pride.

Forty years seem to have gone by in a flash
I'm retired and can relax at last.

Questions for Reflection

Before entering the room of the one you are caring for, take three deep breaths. Allow yourself to clear your mind before stepping through the doorway. Did it make a difference?

Retirement Day
October 21

It's musical chairs being played out today
My morning sacred space has been stolen away.

That's what I get for sleeping in
The most popular seat at the table is given to kin.

The youngest grandson is up for the day
I didn't realize his mom was up and on her way

To catch the last part of her drama series in the bedroom below
She was up so early the sun didn't even show.

The youngest now sitting in my sacred space
Cereal and hot chocolate in place.

Sprinklers are spewing into the neighbor's yard
I asked my daughter to check it; this task was not hard.

The youngest grandson finished his breakfast and settled in her spot
I have my sacred space back for myself—and that means a lot.

Oh, forgot today is my retirement day!
Yippee!

Personal Reflection

When Will My Ship Sail?
October 22

What is true to me
Well, let me see.

The world is upside down, so
What am I going to do? I don't know.

Papers to fill and watch for in the mail
Will it ever stop and let me sail?

Sail into retirement without any fears
Of where my next paycheck will come from; it brings me to tears.

This was not a journey I was planning on
Here it is, and I'm just going along

With the next step and opening the next door
Hoping I don't fall on the floor.

It is exhausting, but a nap is the cure
It helps me clear my head and make rational decisions, I'm sure.

What does the next week bring? Let me see
An exercise expressing what is true to me.

I have stopped the nine-to-five lifestyle
It's time to work on projects I've neglected for a while.

I hope someone will acknowledge my artwork
Find someone to publish my poetry, music, short stories, and book.

Perhaps dig into my hoarded attire
Take it to a thrift store or auction it to the highest buyer.

Spend time with the grandkids and family
A flight down to L.A. to see Mickey.

Travel is on the bucket list, and more
Just release me from this paperwork and watch me soar.

Personal Reflection

Lead Me in the Right Direction
October 23

It has rained and the ground is wet
I admire Mother Nature as the day is set,

The birds are happy they have water to drink
I am happy to sit here and listen to them and think

Oh, today's class will enlighten me on the art of writing in poetic verse
This is what I want to spend my energy on first

For I have poems that twirl in my head
They need to be written down instead.

I have waited a long time to put my ideas in motion
Just lead me in the right direction

To make me a star in the publishing world
I will be forever grateful if you just give me a whirl!

Personal Reflection

Seeking Counsel
October 24

Today is a wonderful day
Time to get up and play.

The birds are up and singing, bringing in a new day
So just a few more moments in my sacred place I will stay

I am excited that one of my projects is materializing
The creation of two songs will be mesmerizing.

A song or two popped in my head some time ago
I wrote them down and felt it was time to go

Into the production lines
With a fabulous song of the times

Only to discover my poem was not a song.

"What?" Yes, there's a difference between the two
I do not listen to music very often, so who knew?

To Google I went to enlighten me
There is a difference, and now I see.

I decided to seek counsel from a younger crowd
Who totally embraced me and made me feel proud.

Today two songs with my poetic verse will be written
For all the world to see.

Personal Reflection

Nerves are Tested
October 25

We are up early, around 4 a.m.
At this time in the morning, I don't know who I am.

Back to sleep for a short little nap
Then up again, the cat in his hammock sack.

The day starts buzzing before my breakfast can be digested
Sometimes this is just how my nerves are tested.

Smooth so far, breakfast and morning chores behind us
Just waiting for Physical Therapist Mike to find us

In rare form and ready to exercise
We announce there has been improvement—he will not be surprised.

Before he comes there is paperwork to ponder
Should I start, or just flounder?

Flounder about and catch up with my chats
Which sounds much more pleasing, so I think I'll do that.

Goodbye for now, I will talk to you soon
Update you on progress with poetry and tunes.

Personal Reflection

CAREGIVER'S POETIC JOURNAL

Patience
October 26

Oh, I forgot you again
Maybe because I was up at 4 a.m. and then

A quick shower, laundry, dishes, and breakfast to eat
Soon our brother-in-law will be here to greet.

Medications delivered and a systematic chart created
All during the distribution of more medications and breakfast—I made it.

More retirement paperwork completed, what a relief
Then on to Instacart, where my brother-in-law will teach—

Teach me how to order from one place or more
Then all you must do is answer the door.

Brother-in-law all settled, ready to take care of you
It is off to the pharmacy to pick up medications, too

But wait. The nurse is at the door
We both go up to the second floor.

We chit chat for a while and when all is done
Off to the pharmacy, oh what fun.

Now back home and exhausted you see
Time for a long nap for me.

Up again and the race begins
Dinner to get ready, medications and then

The decision to take a bath begins
Takes four hours to complete and then laundry all over again.

Time to get ready for bed, you say
I want to finish my journal and stay

Sitting down in my chair to gain strength for the night
Then fix everything up, so all will be right.

Good Night

Personal Reflection

Missing Entry
October 27

Exhausted today, did not write, I will write tomorrow.

Personal Reflection

Season Changing
October 28

Up early to start again
Grandkid is up to celebrate the morning and then

The morning begins and the sun starts to shine
I can hear the geese honking in their line.

It's cold today as fall has sunk in
Soon it will be winter again.

Time for socks and warm woolly sweaters
My choice of the seasons? I think spring would be better.

Now, it is fall and time to take time
To relax and sit in the sacred space that is mine.

Personal Reflection

Losing Control but Staying Strong by Practicing Lovingkindness
OCTOBER 29

I'm not sure what I'm going to write
What is on my mind causes me fright.

I am retired, and these are to be my golden years
The loss of two longtime friends brings me fear

Why did I wait until now and think
This was going to be a magical time, but instead I want to turn to drink.

I had to retire early due to the need to take care of a family member
Who sometimes does not appreciate my help and loses his temper

Over things he has lost control
Over things he does not know.

He questions my every move
Screaming out that a plan of care needs to be improved

Improved so it can be correct each time it is done
Making a simple act of kindness less than fun.

Apology accepted until the next time arises
Unless I can modify my care delivery with disguises.

I know that when he gets stronger
He will be able to manage and will not need my assistance any longer.

In the meantime, I hope we can meet in the middle somewhere
With lovingkindness and show each other we care.

Questions for Reflection

Is your loved one having a difficult time relinquishing control of activities, medications, or treatments? Can you find ways to compromise or help them to feel they have a choice? List them.

Fight the Pain
October 30

The day is over, and I thought we were in the clear
Because of all the extra activity, I fear

You are in pain and do not seem able to rest
This day was a mild day; I would say a test.

A test for the following chemo day
Not sure we're going to make it, but you say

You will try to do so with all your might
I see that in you. I know you will fight.

For now, we will give you a massage, medications, practice deep
breathing, listen to your Sutras and more
To make sure you rest tonight so tomorrow we can get out the door.

Personal Reflection

Respect
NOVEMBER 1

Wow. November already, where has the time gone
It is certain that not all the time has been fun

We were visited many times by Dr Dilaudid, Mrs. Morphine,
and the Decadron twins
When you are up against them, nobody wins.

Simple addition makes me uptight
Counting the next time for pain medication makes us fight.

Your thought process and mathematical skills to you may seem clear
They are not even close, my dear.

To settle the timetable discussion
We developed a medication schedule to teach us a lesson.

Even when under the influence of all those meds
We needn't fight; but respect each other instead.

We need to realize when our friends come to call
To respect each other's options, large ones and small.

Personal Reflection

Exhaustion
November 2

Oh, my November 2
What do you do?

No sleep for the night and had to think
Passed out while I sat, just to get a wink.

Coffee helps to keep my eyes awake
Not sure if that assures I won't make a mistake

One mistake in deciding, or two
I think today will be a quiet one to stay with you.

One chore of the day will be to check on our investment
We have a meeting today and hope I'll know how my money will be spent.

It's important to know and calculate the retirement days
So I have enough money to survive and play.

Personal Reflection

Take a Deep Breath to Breathe in a New Day
November 3

Amazing when I look out from my sacred place
No lights on anywhere across the fence in that space

Which is usually slightly lit
Not very much now, it's too early.

Not early for us, 6:50 a.m. We were up before
I'm not sure; it was shortly after four.

Too dark to see across the way
I finally hear the traffic rolling, I have to say

All the house noise I am creating inside
Prevents me from hearing the world outside.

Hot water boiling and a load of laundry going
Says the day is starting, so I better get moving.

Physical therapy, home health nurse, grandkids to visit
A little more time in my sacred space—just a minute

To take a deep breath to bring in a new day
Relax, rejuvenate for this is the Caritas way.

Personal Reflection

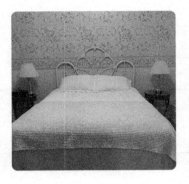

Nap Time
NOVEMBER 4

Missed a day, no time to think, but able to have a nap
and sleep for a while during the night.

CAREGIVER'S POETIC JOURNEY

Personal Reflection

A Thankful Reflection
November 7

Another day and here we are
No time for my sacred space so far.

Gobbled my food and here we go
A full day ahead—just go with the flow.

Even though the day is rough
I can reflect on what I am thankful for, but it is tough.

Yesterday was fun; I had time to meet
With my artistic group of nurse companions, which was sweet.

We shared upcoming projects and treasured time together
Then back to reality and feeling better

The rejuvenation did not stop there
It was nap time, so up the stairs

A two-hour nap quieted the mind
Which soon gave me energy to complete the chores left behind.

Today is another one of those busy days
A doctor's appointment and MRI.

We make it through the video call
Then rush to be ready to walk down the hall

To the stairs and out to the car
Then to the hospital for the MRI. And so far,

Everything is going smoothly until we get to the admitting desk
The receptionist announces the price of the test.

Well, I guess the COBRA I paid for had not found its way through
The receptionist says a thousand-dollar co-pay is due.

As I gasp and want to faint on the floor
The receptionist says Member Services can help. They are on the same floor.

Off to the MRI you go and next we will see
What Member Services will say about the fee.

Personal Reflection

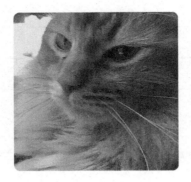

Time is Not Mine
November 9

I am exhausted and you ask why
"Because I am running around," I will not lie.

Up and down the stairs I go
Until I am in pain from head to toe

But for a moment I have some time
To put up my feet, a moment which is mine!

It did not last long.

Personal Reflection

Missing Entries
NOVEMBER 10 - NOVEMBER 22

Sometimes life is chaotic, and you do not even have time to journal, so some days were missed.

Personal Reflection

Returning
November 23

Sorry old friend that I left you behind
I convinced myself I did not have time

To write down a word or two
Or just spend some time talking to you.

Much to do though so much has been done
Many of the tasks have not been fun.

I've been exhausted dealing with retirement papers
I hope eventually it will all taper

I can enjoy time with family and friends
That type of joy I hope will never end.

Personal Reflection

Thanksgiving Surprise
NOVEMBER 24

I am tired but let me see
What am I thankful for and how did I spend Thanksgiving?

I spent it together with the one I love
We spent a quiet day together and watched the Macy's Day Parade;
that was fun.

As we genuinely enjoyed a nontraditional meal
We pondered what was going to be our next, and how did we feel

About disturbing the family to make something fresh
As you know, their culinary skills are the best.

We had a few meals in the freezer, we knew
Just enough for a day or two.

After pondering together, we fell sound asleep
Not a sound could be heard, not even a peep.

Suddenly, a knock was heard from the downstairs front door
Guess what? It was the family with more—

More food for the rest of the week
We could enjoy every bite, oh what a feast.

I am thankful, so grateful for all that was given
This was truly one of the finest Thanksgivings.

Questions for Reflection

Have you had your cup of tea or coffee, hydrated with water, brushed your teeth, and taken a shower? Did someone bring you and your loved one a special treat?

Blessings
November 25

One more holiday has come and gone
Not sure who played in the football game or who won

We did soak in a movie or two
Enjoyed closing our eyes and taking a snooze.

I also enjoyed the antics of cat, squirrel and more
Which carried on until I shut the patio door.

In between naps we ate like kings and queens
Now it is night, marking the end, it seems.

Simba the Cat has the job of guarding our home
He protects us from his throne.

Tonight, his throne is at the end of the bed. He is perched up high
Stretched out comfortably, he closes his eyes.

As we all are relaxed and the night ends, it is time to reflect
On the blessings we have and the ones we have not experienced yet.

Personal Reflection

Spread Lovingkindness Through My Writings and Poetry
NOVEMBER 26

What I have discovered today will make you smile
I've been pondering what my end project will be for a while.

I have had so many irons in the fire
Most of the flames grow dim; some expire.

Two songs to hit the golden stage
Or maybe only part of my book of wonders and I'll need to turn the page.

Wait, an idea popped into my head
They usually do when I'm sound asleep in bed.

I will still count on my songs to be produced
My journal will be my masterpiece and you my muse

You really have come aboard to see the real me
To join me in my mission to spread lovingkindness through my writings and poetry.

I'm amazed we're connecting so strongly in this quest
To shine above the stars—to make it our best.

Into the next chapter in life, we will journey
Together with each other in peace and harmony.

Personal Reflection

Gratitude Through Music
November 27

I attended a class about music and how it captures your
mind, body, and soul
How rhythm influences both young and old.

I shared one of my songs
We had several sing-a-longs.

It was a fabulous day
Thank you in every way.

Thank you, Mary, Kathy, and my new artistic friends
Good night now as my journal entry ends.

Personal Reflection

Exhausting Day of Challenges
November 28

My phone battery needs recharging and so does my computer
I wish that my battery could be recharged by going to bed sooner.

Here I am reflecting on our exhausting day of challenges
A trip to the hospital for chemo treatment and the pharmacy;
that's how it is.

Hopefully, tomorrow there will be nothing on the agenda
Except a phone call or two and cuddling up with a warm
blanket in our hacienda.

Now time to rest my head
My eyes are almost shut, so I'm heading for bed.

Good night, my dear friend, I will see you in the morning.

Questions for Reflection

Dream on, You Say
November 29

November 29
Lookin' fine.

Today I accomplished another website task
I think I might be getting used to this at last.

Dream on, you say
It's the best of hopes and wishes which may.

A pile of papers, now up to my knees
I hope to have time to organize them—please!

Social Security is taking its time
HR Retirement Services said they will not leave me behind

Until my benefits are all settled in place
Then I can start moving at a slower pace.

Then more time to sit at your bedside, not as stressed
Since all this will be behind me; oh, what a mess.

I am taking twenty minutes to relax downstairs
Settle the cat and make sure I take care

Of all the last-minute chores and wrap up the night
Then crawl in bed and turn out the light.

Questions for Reflection

Wintertime

November 30

Oh boy, winter is here, it is toasty inside
Hopefully, we can slip into the covers soon and hide.

Questions for Reflection

The Importance of Communication
December 1

This journal is so appropriate to how I feel
My feet have been walking so hard they're beginning to peel.

I thought all your requests had been made tonight
I sat down in my chair, thinking all was right

You stated you wanted to go to sleep
I packed up my gear and was on my feet.

You had me turn back for a few chosen chores
I just looked at you and started to roar.

As we finished those couple of demands
I thought this type of communication was getting out of hand.

I explained to you at last that I was tired
I was going to bed, and this was my last task.

You explained you were trying to settle yourself down
Wouldn't need to get up from the bed and wouldn't make a sound.

We laughed together as the cat strolled by
I said the cat knew differently, and I gave out a sigh.

We acknowledged that things didn't go as they should
Now back in bed we understood

The importance of communication versus a fight
We hugged each other and said good night.

Questions for Reflection

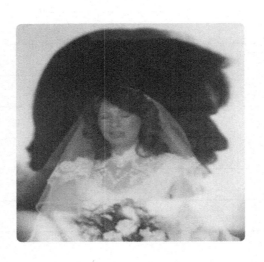

CAREGIVER'S POETIC JOURNEY

Loss of a Great Person

January 10th, 2024, would have been our 43rd wedding anniversary but I lost my husband to metastatic mesothelioma on December 30, 2023. We fought the battle for over eleven years, and he hung on until he knew I was financially stable and had family to provide for my emotional needs.

Over the last six months his health had declined, but we still went to his chemotherapy sessions and modified our lifestyle to anticipate the next diet change, the next piece of equipment needed, etc. I even retired early, because I didn't know how I could care for him and work full time.

The family was here to help with meals, transportation, moral support, entertainment (grandkids), and to be by his side. I had just signed up for Mary Rockwood Lane's class, (forty education hours) and was finishing twenty-six hours of another course when we ended up in the emergency room.

I stayed by his side and when he was asleep, I would listen to my courses. Each course provided insight on how to be a loving, kind, empathetic caregiver. Shortly after we came home from the hospital and started home health, he showed signs of side effects from chemotherapy and a decline in his health. He was on Doxorubicin: the "Red Devil." His skin was turning from red to purple, became very thin, and tore when he lifted himself up in bed. He had mouth sores, and we thought shingles had returned, this time in his nose and throat. He had trouble swallowing. Even with antivirals, antibiotics, and morphine for pain, he was not able to recover.

We struggled to know if we would be financially stable because I'd just turned sixty-five and needed to sign up for social security and Medicare. To switch over to a retirement health care plan, Medicare A and B had to be in place. My health insurance was on and then off again because they could not get the paperwork straight. I was on the phone all day in between caring for Muhammad's needs.

We were able to settle things down and have a quiet Christmas together (daughter and grandkids included), and he presented me with an engraved iPad, the latest model, so I could store my poetry and stories. He admitted to me that he realized why I followed the practices and teaching of Jean's theory of Caring Science. He'd happened to watch one of my continuing education sessions and realized other nurses followed this same path and they too found peace, joy, equanimity, and solace in Jean's words of wisdom. My family had been coming to the house while I attended Mary's course where I explored my artistic expression. Sometimes it revealed thoughts and feelings I didn't know I had.

Mary encouraged us to write a journal, and this book was born, to be titled *Caregiver's Poetic Journal*. This was to be published as a forty-five-page journal with the daily poems I created while caring for my husband—but it did not end there. The last entry in the first chapter was about the importance of communicating with each other. Shortly after the end of the class he declined greatly, and I did not want him to pass away at home.

I wanted one more chance to keep him alive. He agreed to be taken to the hospital. We called 911 and he was carried down the stairs to the ambulance. The doctor gave him only twenty-four hours to live, but he rallied for a few more days. Family and friends came to see him, and he was coherent enough to talk with them. Even the day before he died, we watched his favorite show and listened to his Surahs.

I fell into a deep sleep for the first time and woke to find him less responsive. I called the family because his oxygen level was dropping, and his heart rate was elevated. They provided him with oxygen and comfort care. The family prayed over him, and he was able to say his last prayer. His sisters said he was looking around the room and at the door before he took his last breath. He soon passed, and the family made the arrangements to have him sent to the funeral home so they could wash and wrap him before placing him in his final resting place.

When I saw him for the last time, he had a smile on his face (which was not there when he passed away), his lips were plump and the sores in his nose were gone, though the sores had not been artificially removed or covered with makeup. We had over two hundred family and friends attend the service with only a few hours' notice.

Women could attend the burial site but could only look on at a distance. The men opened the gravesite by hand; they processed around him, praying for him, and then they lowered him into the ground. Every person at the gravesite added soil until it was full. Family and friends gathered for three days to pray, and gathered again, several more times.

Since then, he has come to me several times in my dreams, once to tell me to get up, get out of bed and get dressed, and another time he snuggled up against me and I woke thinking he was there. I know in my heart he is resting and is no longer in pain and I can accept this and cherish the fact that he is in heaven, but my body has a different idea, which may take a while to overcome.

   I am so thankful for all who have comforted me and my family. The next chapter in my life's journey will not be an easy one without the patriarch of the family, but I will carry on his legacy and pass the history of his greatness to generations to come.

PART TWO

Light in
the Universe

CAREGIVER'S POETIC JOURNAL

A Day of Firsts
February 26

A Day of Firsts
As your journey in life changes, you may experience a day of firsts.

First day without a loved one, so you shed tears
Health is changing and now you're in fear.

Need to travel outside your comfort zone
Wishing you were back home even though you're alone.

Time to think, time to reflect
What life will show you, what will be next.

Time to reach out to the ones you love
You'll have support to carry on.

As life brings on new challenges you will learn
That God will be blessing you with each twist and turn.

Today is another day to recall the firsts without you.

As my journey of caretaker ended
I was not so aware of all the things I didn't know—

Know now or even remember
We had been sheltered for years, you and me.

COVID and cancer locked us inside
Striving each day for a miracle to stay alive.

Sheltered from dining and shopping and then
Sheltered from outside family and friends.

It didn't seem enough to shelter
Your time had come, and you had to leave me.

As I tap on my phone to send this message out
A tear forms and I want to shout.

These days of firsts are exhausting to me
I wish you were here to watch and see

The roads are the same, but I forgot how to get around
The trees have grown bigger, and more buildings sprung from the ground.

The items in the store are locked up
Might be inconvenient but looks orderly and clean

I went to church for the first time alone
Several years I celebrated mass by phone.

There will be many more firsts without you, I know
Family and friends will be there to show—

Show and guide me on the right things to do
As I accomplish new firsts, first times without you.

Questions for Reflection

Take a moment to reflect on how you are feeling. Use this time to identify those observations or feelings and use your journal to capture your thoughts.

Words are Left Behind
February 27

Pardon me, journal
I already forgot about you.

Yesterday's thoughts rolled through my head
Instead of writing I rehearsed them instead.

I already know that was a mistake to do
When the thoughts are out of my head, we are through.

The moment has passed with the words left behind
Then I must contemplate a new rhyme in my mind.

LIGHT IN THE UNIVERSE

Personal Reflection

Honoring the Nurses
February 28

Another day without you but as you see
Simba and I are in our sacred morning space.

You're in our minds and in our hearts
As we start a new day in the dark.

We're up early like we would be with you
Now it will only be us two.

Up early as the juices are flowing
While others are tucked in their warm beds snoring.

Up early today to sit in my sacred place
To jot in my journal early, just in case

These thoughts are forgotten again; for throughout the day
As I recite them in my mind, they slip away.

So, let us begin with what occurred yesterday
It was a magical, marvelous day for me.

I gathered trinkets, treasures, and gifts
To honor the nurses who helped us

During those times when we struggled, those last hours of time
The last hours of time, yours, and mine.

We will honor you by giving back to them
Everything they did for us and then

I will share with others the gifting we have done
Then others can do the same, to comfort themselves
after losing a loved one.

Personal Reflection

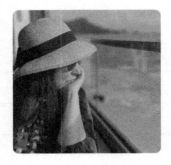

What a State I am in
February 29

I don't know where to begin
To tell you the state I'm in.

Surprised you, indeed
It is not a state of mind, but the state of Hawaii!

My daughter has cared for me since you passed
And we decided to venture out at last.

After a day in the sun and sand at my feet
I'm in a comfortable hotel room, ready to sleep.

We received a beautiful lei when we arrived
And when we are done adorning them, we will not set them aside.

We'll place the flowers back into nature
In your honor we will float them out to sea.

Or make a sea turtle out of the sand
And place them around it and then

Say a prayer in your honor, just before we depart
This magical land which I now hold close to my heart.

Personal Reflection

A Bigger Bond Has Been Made
March 1

Is it March? How time passes by!

It seems like just yesterday I was with you
Wondering and thinking what we needed to do.

To keep the sunshine and energy in our lives
As we struggled through our challenges alive.

I'm out there in the real world again
Sometimes think I'm only flopping in the wind,

As I stand on the sands of Waikiki
I cannot think of anything else but what you mean to me.

Sophia and I have explored half the island
Sometimes I need to stop here and then

Off to another adventure for the next day
Everything should be in order, they say.

It is a beautiful sight to see
I know you are enjoying it with me.

Tomorrow is the last day
On this magnificent island where we've stayed.

You will be happy to know of the deeper bond we've made
As we spent the many hours and played

Played with the dolphins, splashed in the water and more
Swimming, waterfalls, hiking, shopping, fireworks—my feet are sore.

Tomorrow is another day
Good night from Sophia and me.

Personal Reflection

Grateful For Endless Treasures
March 2

Majestic beauty, frolic in the ocean blue
Something dear to my heart, and true.

What a gorgeous world we live in
Cultures too many to count with the strokes of a pen.

All united in one
Striving for life and liberty.

All watching the waves and admiring the view
Amazing what God has given to me and you.

Go out each day with your head held up high
Be thankful, be grateful for all you have inside

Inside your mind, your heart, and soul
We are here only once, and we are not alone.

To enjoy God's endless treasures as far as we can see
Pull up your pant legs, roll up your sleeves

Take a dive in the blue ocean with me.

Personal Reflection

A Cultural Connection
March 3 and March 4

A two-day project! Inspired from my trip to Hawaii just a day ago.
Talofa: Samoan for hello
Tofa: Samoan for goodbye: hope we will meet again sometime
Fa'afetai: Samoan for thank you: thank you for a wonderful time.
Aloha: Hawaiian for hello and goodbye
Mahalo: Hawaiian for thank you: our time has ended, so we give a great sigh
I will always remember what rich culture you have shared, my Ohana
About you, your history, traditions, culture, food, and dress, truly "Nirvana."
Malo e Lelei: Tonga for hello
Nofo a: Tonga for goodbye
Malo aupito: Tonga for thank you very much.
Your cultural heritage you dance and sing aloud
A nation so strong and proud.
Ia ora na: Tahitian for hello
Nana: Tahitian for goodbye: I hope we will forever keep in touch
Mauruuru roa: Tahitian for thank you very much.
Bula: Fijian for a casual hello
Moce: Fijian informal goodbyes: to an island with water so blue
Vinaka vakalevu: Fijian for thank you: thank you, we hope someday to visit you.
Kia ora: Aotearoa for hello
Haere r : Aotearoa for goodbye: for now, we need to dash
Kia Ora: Aotearoa for thank you: we'll remember this trip;
we wished it would forever last
Thank you all for welcoming us into your family, your heart
Thank you for the (HA) you showed us from the start
Maika'i ke ola a me ka pōmaika'i iā 'oukou a pau
Good life and blessings to you all
Merci beaucoup from Mom's side of the family
Mòran taing from Dad's side of the family
Shukriya from my husband's side of the family
May the breath and circle of life (HA) forever feed our lungs, open our hearts, brighten our minds, and lift our souls to spread the transpersonal beacons of light to everyone we meet, enlightening all, making this a universal love which will glow for all to feel and see forever.
Mahalo

Personal Reflection

A New Adventure in Creativity
MARCH 5

Entry nine
And I am fine

As I expressed in another entry, I wrote that I planned to be adventurous with my creativity
I sat in my sacred place and dove into a new activity.

I had just watched *Moana* and remembered my adventure to Hawaii, so I gathered my box of jewelry-making supplies, beads, strings, and shells. Soon the juices were flowing like a rush and the following was created:

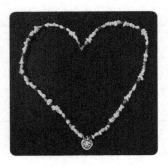

Personal Reflection

Forgiveness
MARCH 6

Entry ten, forgot again
Went to bed early and

Realized an entry had not been done
Tomorrow will be another day, so I can create one.

Personal Reflection

Wishing You Were with Me
March 7

Entry eleven
I am in heaven

Sitting near the window in a spot of sun
Comfortable and warm, my day's just begun.

I slept for hours with dreams so wild
I even dreamt my friend had another child.

I needed the rest
My body knows best.

The day before I was sitting at the kitchen table going through the mail
Fell asleep right in the pile.

Afraid I might throw something important away
I gave up my chore for another day.

That day is today but still moving at the pace of a sloth
I need to tackle the bills and laundry to reduce its growth.

I'll just go on with a pace that's natural to me
Until I'm ready to increase the speed.

Not sure when that will be
I continue to stop and wish you were here with me.

It can be lonely and so quiet in this place
Family, friends, and Simba help fill up the space.

Miss you greatly!

Personal Reflection

The Bread of Life
March 8

The Bread of Life is Joy and Gratitude

When you think of the bread of life what do you think of
Do you think about the mana that fell from the heavens above?

What comes to mind, what do you feel inside
Do you think of survival, or does it paint a bright picture in your mind?

Do you feel joy and gratitude
What's bestowed on you?

What is one thing you can say
You're thankful for this day?

In God's grand plan
We don't always know what's at hand

The mysteries and journeys we will take
The ones that will be present for us when we wake

Awake to the many gifts that the bread of life will bring
To me, to you, the universe, let us shout and sing

Amen

Personal Reflection

Intimate Moments
March 9

Oh my, I am tired but so proud
Of what my daughter and I have done.

Thank you for this time together, to bond and share
Intimate moments to show we care

We cleaned her kitchen and threw out old stuff
Then ran to the store to replace it all, but that wasn't enough

We continued to clean and place out all our new treasures
Sophia was worn out first, but I still found pleasure

In throwing out the old and bringing in the new
Finding trivial things that might give pleasure to me and you.

It's time to wind down and turn off the energy for now
The thought of getting out of bed in the morning makes me frown.

We will carry on and the morning will shine
As we look 'round and know we've left the dust bunnies behind.

Personal Reflection

Happy Heavenly Birthday
March 10

Happy heavenly birthday to the one I love
I feel your warmth, your smile, your presence from above.

I woke up early after a cleaning party at your daughter's house
Much to remove and luckily, no sighting of a mouse.

You'd be proud that we accomplished our goal
Managed to go out to lunch and then the mall.

I didn't realize this had been another first for me
Going to a mall after sheltering in place during COVID... finally free.

We came home and she fell asleep
While I tidied up and made that last sweep.

As the last chore was completed, I felt so grateful for the time we had together
The accomplishments we achieved could not have been better.

Up the next morning to see what we'd achieved
Had a small breakfast, then time to flee

From Stockton to Sacramento, I did go
My goal was to be on time for church and so

I hit the freeway and away I went
Made it in time, truly blessed.

I waited for the mass to begin; I noticed the date on the marquee
It was March 10, and I wished you a happy heavenly birthday.

I held back the tears and carried on
It was not easy; this was a difficult one

A difficult first in the many to come
I am strong and will conquer each one.

I also went up in line
To receive a blessing for the first time

The fear of COVID had held me behind
Today I challenged my fear and waited for a sign.

A sign that it was safe to join others, you know
A sign from you giving me the green light to go.

Even now when those first-time challenges appear
You will be there to support me and show me a sign

Thank you and happy heavenly birthday to the one I love
Thank you for being there for me, watching out for me
from the heavens above.

Personal Reflection

My Work is Dedicated to You
March 11

Am I a poetry hoarder? We will see
I have poems written on paper, in books, notes in the phone,
computers, laptops, you tell me!

That's okay. I know
There are many poetic pieces out there, ready to show.

Show the world how rhythmic verse
Allows for self-expression, which should always come first.

First for self, let the thoughts flow free
Then they can be shared for all to see.

Simple rhymes are created from thoughts in the mind
The rest flows in writing form, in time.

Writing poetry is my passion
It's important to keep my treasures in orderly fashion.

I have not used your tablet yet to store all my works
This will be my next challenge—to defeat all the quirks.

The challenge will be to learn how to upload them in the iPad
you dedicated to me
The one place they will all be present for me to see.

I will be able to assemble them to be published, this is the plan
Which will be easier now that I'm retired, with more time on my hands.

My work will be dedicated to you, wait and see
They will be gifts of remembrance; a dedication to you from me.

Personal Reflection

Writer's Block
MARCH 12

Missed again
Nothing in my head

As I work through the days
I hope to write my thoughts and what I want to say

In my journal, so a poem might appear
Sad to say I missed another day.

Personal Reflection

When We First Met

March 13

Where is the time going? I don't know
The months are passing, not slow.

Today is another day, so we'll see
What opportunities will open for me.

To begin with, I'm entertained by the cat
I'm not sure what has gotten into him.

He just ran into the patio screen
I wonder if it's a squirrel he's seen

Perched on the windowsill
He feels protected. He is patient and still.

He's my main companion now that you are gone
We have our routines, some short, some long.

Up early in the morning like it used to be
When caring for you, the cat and me.

We sit in our sacred spot
Giving time to write, sometimes not a lot.

An entry here and there
Just a record of what I'm thankful for and what I can bear

Some days and nights are lonely, but we carry on
With you etched in our memory like a pleasant song.

Miss you and wish you were here
Like in the olden days that I hold so dear

I know you're in a more heavenly place
Don't forget to save me a space

Close to you and close to your heart
Like when we first met, from the very start.

Personal Reflection

On a Do-Nothing Day
March 14

What do you do on a do-nothing day?

What do you do on a do-nothing day?
Sleep past noon is one way

To spend the day in comfortable clothes
Not sure if I will step outside; well, that's how it goes

On a do-nothing day!

The wind is blustery as it whips through the trees
It looks like a day when indoors will be right for me.

I'm not interested in making any business calls
Tomorrow will come quickly; then I'll bundle them all.

For now, it's time to kick back without pain
No rushing around like I'm insane.

Just a very pleasant call from my friend far away
As she says good night and I start my day.

The cat needs attention. It's time for a belly rub
Time to chase his toy mouse and stare out the patio screen door.

Not too much action will we be seeing today
As we kick back and relax on our do-nothing day!

Questions for Reflection

*How have you practiced lovingkindness for yourself today?
Have you taken time to have a cup of tea or walk outside?*

On a Do-Something Day
March 15

Up early, usually to a pitter-patter of little feet
Four to be exact, up to greet

The rising sun in all its glory,
But Simba's in his hammock and snoring

Those happy little paws must be slow today
For me, it's a do-something day

Yesterday I just lounged around
Didn't accomplish much, but I found

I was more relaxed than I have been before
I slept through the night, which I adore.

A great sleep, and now some energy to burn
Let's see how productive I'll be, and what rewards I'll earn.

That feeling of fulfillment when a task is complete
Let's see what I'll accomplish and then I will treat

Myself to an evening of relaxation
Cuddle up to my four-footed companion and a soft, soft cushion.

Read a book or watch TV tomorrow—we'll wait and see
What exciting adventures will be bestowed on me.

Personal Reflection

Reminiscing With a Friend
March 16

Kids made it home from their trip, as you see
They ransacked the house, if you could believe

After we spent hours cleaning, plus a professional as well
Sophia picked up after them as far as I could tell.

I didn't worry; I was out with a friend
We gossiped and then

Went out to dinner for soup and a shake
I came back home and could hardly stay awake.

Before she left, we discussed our next Caring Science project to present
For the international conference; this will be our best one yet!

Personal Reflection

Miracle World

March 17

I don't live in a material world
I live in a miracle world.

My life is one exciting world of miracles, a world where
possibilities never end
To cherish, to hold, and to believe in.

For the greatness you (Muhammad) gave in your lifetime
Has, in the many kindnesses you bestowed,
come back in miracles, ten-fold.

From the well you built in Ghana that replenishes many
To all you reached out to, especially family

I see every day and, in my dreams,
What you meant to the world and what you meant to me.

I struggle hard to spread caring and lovingkindness for all to see
You opened yourself, eyes and heart, at the end to show you always
believed in me.

I thank you so much for this magnificent gift
Which we'll share with others and as we lift—

Lift our hearts to our marvelous healthcare caregivers, such a loving,
caring, comforting, extraordinary team
We thank you all and Julie for completing this last journey of
thankfulness and gratefulness beyond our wildest dreams.

Julie, MSN, RN,CCRN, CNL, Caritas Nurse®, Clinical Practice Consultant Adult Services and Care was instrumental in providing our gift basket donation to the team of healthcare providers who took care of us during Muhammad's last days in the hospital.

Personal Reflection

Need to Remember to Center Myself
March 18

What can I say, I missed out again on writing my thoughts during the morning sunrise. A day must not start out in such a hurry that I forget about centering myself before heading out the door or starting a project.

Personal Reflection

Commemorating You
March 19

A new beginning could be in store
If I just take a moment to open the door,

Peek inside my world of possibilities
Something might spark my interest and intrigue me

To work on a project or two
I have several in mind to commemorate you.

Some are still in the planning stage
One has sprouted wings and has already been made

We have spread smiles on the nurses and staff
Who were there to assist us when they passed

Passed your door in the last days when you held your head up high
Before we all wept and said our goodbyes.

Love you!

Personal Reflection

The Road is Not a Road; it is a Journey
March 20

Something I wrote in the last class

The road is not a road; it is a journey
One that sometimes takes us on a path when we are alone

As we quietly assess the softness of the sand
We find there is another to take our hand

To lift us, to guide us, to show us the way
The journey will not be so lonely that day.

"Namaste"

Yesterday was my first day to go to the grocery store by
myself after four years of isolation from caring for my husband
with cancer and during COVID. I also went to
my first open confessional service.

Dedicated to Saint Kim Agi Agatha

Personal Reflection

The Scarf Dance
March 21

The Scarf Dance will be dedicated to you
The colors are so magnificent, so blue.

Colors of the ocean will flow in the wind
As the congregation enters the room, the magic begins.

As the music flows, the scarves gently twirl
More will participate and give it a whirl

The body, mind, and spirit flow free
As we meditate on what we are grateful to see.

Smiles will light up the ballroom
As we demonstrate how the body can destress

As we take part in this blessed event
We remember why giving is important and what it meant

To you as you graced so many during your life
Being there, stretching out a hand, making all right.

As the scarves of the ocean take flight
I'll look at the crowd and admire smiles so bright.

Again, this is time to say thank you, for you are the one
We are so grateful for what you have done.

Personal Reflection

If Our Sacred Places Could Tell a Story
March 22

If our sacred places could tell a story
About what makes our hearts shine in all their glory

It can be intricate with trinkets of old
Or a simple place to sit, dine, and hold

A holding place where you can be inspired in time
To write something magical, something to rhyme.

It might be a place where you've gathered candles, scents,
a picture of your firstborn
Objects that connect you to the past.

No need to seek them out for they are there
They are the everyday places where you share—

Share and reminisce about stories of life and thoughts true
Sharing the deepest parts and history of you.

Questions for Reflection

What have you done to brighten your journaling room? Are the doors open? Do you have fresh air? Tell about the special space you have and how this space rejuvenates you.

Ocean Meditation
March 23

Imagine yourself strolling on the beach on a bright summer's day, the warm sand beneath your toes
You can feel a mild breeze coming off the ocean
This makes you feel at ease.

The clouds, like puffs of cotton, slowly drift by
While your heart beats with the pulsating rhythm of the ocean's waves
As you stroll along the oceanside or relax on its sandy beach.

Now: take a moment and be still
Savor those feelings and take three deep breaths.
Wrap your heart with your breath
And reflect on where you are in this moment

Shift your thoughts to what you are grateful for, what brings you joy and happiness.
Breathe deeply three more times.
Now extend your gratitude, joy, happiness, and love to the universe.

Personal Reflection

Embrace Each Moment
March 24

Embrace each moment before that moment passes you by

Capture it in journal, picture, painting, poem, or dance
Make sure this moment is preserved forever, make sure it is stored.

These captured moments can fill your heart with gladness
or reveal a wound that needs to heal
By bringing out your artistic talents, your feelings,
your healing will be revealed.

Maybe not at first will you see what message is present
By capturing the moment it will be time well spent

I have captured moments so dear to me
They will be forever present rather than a mist of my life's history.

I offer you this blossoming lotus of wisdom, lovingkindness,
gratefulness, and joy
You can learn to embrace those moments, providing you
extra time to toy

With the inner most meaning, the miraculous message
you've created from the heart
An artistic expression, that precious moment, captured in your art.

LIGHT IN THE UNIVERSE

Personal Reflection

Nurturing My Singing Voice
March 25

We were up early before the sun thought to rise
It was just me and the cat who fell back to sleep; I was surprised.

I spent most of the day going through papers and old emails
Figuring out what was important to keep. Got tired,
but felt I would prevail.

Stopped for a brief time for an enlightening class with Mary
Where I reconnected with my singing voice, which was hairy.

I have not been singing or taking part
In a singing group, I just recently participated in church, for a start.

I used to sing and harmonize
It had been a long sabbatical from singing, I realized.

Today I took the plunge and rediscovered my vocal range
It was hard at first and felt very strange.

The exercise opened my breath, my heart, my voice
Now when I want to express myself, I have a choice.

When next Sunday rolls around and I'm sitting in the pew
I have the choice to belt out the songs, so I'm heard by not only me,
but by you!

LIGHT IN THE UNIVERSE

Personal Reflection

Place of Honor
MARCH 26

Can you imagine, this should have been #30's place of honor, but I was too lazy to make an entry.

Personal Reflection

A Poetic Verse from Me to You
March 27

I'd better make an entry before I forget once more
Or feel like I have no time and run out the door.

What a joke that last verse can be
All I want to do is stay home, just me.

Not sure where the motivation and energy has been hidden
all these years
My reserve may not be found again

I face a table of undone work that should matter to me
When I look at it, all I want to do is sleep.

What did I do this morning? I hardly dare to tell
I pressed the print button on my last journal book's entry, and

Forty or more papers have been printed to be on the table
At least it is together and does not need to be labeled.

If I quickly place it in my last journal book in an orderly fashion
I will feel complete, accomplished, for I have preserved my passion—

My passion to communicate in poetic verse
Sometimes at my best and sometimes at my worst.

A day should not go by without a word or two
A poetic verse from me to you.

Personal Reflection

Faced with Another First Without You
March 28

Number thirty-two; what do you do
When faced with another first without you?

While filling out a questionnaire
It asks for your marital status. If you dare

To mark the appropriate space
Where your status is now "widow," oh, what a state.

Your mind races, your heart gives a squeeze
It's not something to take lightly.

This will continue from time to time
New firsts will pop up and sometimes you pay them no mind.

But the big events like holidays and special occasions hit you hard
It will be important not to be alarmed

You will make it through, for you are strong
Your family, friends, and faith will be there to help you along.

LIGHT IN THE UNIVERSE

Personal Reflection

The Greatest Gift
March 29

Lazy today
Just wanted to play.

Be creative—and that is what I did
But I took some time to reflect like I should.

Reflect on the life you gave us this day, Jesus
When they nailed you to the cross and then took you away

To a tomb where they anointed you with oil
Paying homage to you, for you prevailed.

You rose from the tomb Easter morn
All of us are grateful and want to adorn

Ourselves with our favorite attire, off to church we go
To thank you for the greatest gift you gave us, the greatest gift
we will ever know.

Personal Reflection

My World of Artistic Expression
March 30

Journal entry for today: talking about art supplies that I gathered at the beginning of Mary's programs and where I am today. I am truly blessed on how Mary's spiritual guidance and wisdom have opened my world of artistic expression.

My New Wooden Toolbox of Art Supplies

A new wooden toolbox of wonderment before my very eyes
Like a carpenter, I have many tools, and I can use them to magically paint the skies.

Skies of white, skies of blue
A rainbow or two.

Today would be a cloudy one; it is raining outside
We gaze though the patio door at Mother Nature's wonders from inside—

Inside the walls of our comfortable home
Where I sit in my sacred space, but I am not alone.

Simba is experiencing limited screen time right now
The door to his world has been temporarily closed, meow!

The rain will eventually stop, the clouds will drift away
Then screen time will be reopened; it will be time to play.

Personal Reflection

Happy Easter
March 31

Happy Easter!

Made it to church and bellowed the words to all the songs
I really started to feel like I belong.

It had been some time since I had been in a crowd
Approximately 1,400 people. I did not know that was allowed.

They sat in different sections and even outside on a pew
While we sat comfortably inside where there was a better view.

They scurried in as the hour drew near
Then we would all be together to listen to the story so dear,

The story of how Christ rose from the dead
When they opened his tomb, all that was left were wrappings: threads.

The story continues to let us all know
That our Lord suffered, died, was buried, and then rose—

Rose from this earth to be with his Father
Paving the way for us who come after.

Amen and thank you!

Questions for Reflection

*Take a moment to reflect on what you are grateful for.
During this time, be open to the mysteries and the unknown which have graced your path during this journey.*

Another First
April 1

I had a short thought tonight: I had a lovely day and was very productive
Even sang a song in front of a small audience.

Another one of those firsts
Many more will be out there for me.

Right now, I am happy to say
I am tucked nicely and warmly in my bed and that's where
I'm going to stay.

Good night, everyone.

Personal Reflection

A Chill Down My Spine
April 2

April two
How do you do?

I have a new poem entry for you
Poem created after communicating with Anne in
"The Art of Nursing" blog.

A Chill Down My Spine
Energy to heal, energy to feel well
The rejuvenation so mighty that we must tell.

All who are touched, they all will find
When the Caritas touch has been felt, the feeling is divine.

Personal Reflection

A Strawberry Éclair if You Dare
April 3

A strawberry éclair if you dare
For breakfast, for self-care.

An indulgence so fine
I can only call mine.

No calories were spared
On this fine day of self-care.

Sometimes it is simply great fun to indulge!

Personal Reflection

Poetry and Affirmation
April 4

Today is a new day
We are on our way.

First, I will sit at the table and open my eyes
Digest my breakfast, and then I will dive

Into my paperwork and poetry
We are up early, the cat and I, so much productive work ahead of me.

I have some great ideas, ways to gather my written words
Affirmations that will stir—

Stir emotions: joy, gratitude, happiness, and sadness
Bubbling with ideas I didn't know I had.

I will say good morning and goodbye for now
The surge of ideas is running, and I must figure out how

I will be able to write them in time
With the continuous thought that my time should be mine.

Goodbye for now and I hope I may
Have enough energy to put my ideas into motion today.

Personal Reflection

Grateful for Tomorrow
April 5

In bed with a pillow under my head

With Simba the Cat by my side
Too tired today even to rhyme.

I've been lazy with my journal for the last week
It is time to refocus and show

That I am still taking a moment out of my life
To reflect, be grateful, and ponder what the next day will be like.

Will I venture out, will I complete a new task
I am not one to pace myself, but this will not last.

Lessons are learned sometimes at a slow rate
I am sure I will come to an understanding of how I must pace—

Pace out my time, pace out a chore
There will always be tomorrow, a tomorrow to explore.

Personal Reflection

Release of Tears, Self-Healing
April 6

As I sit here in my sacred space
Bundled up and tears running down my face,

This is what they say may happen anytime, anyplace.

I looked for my "Ocean" presentation and a picture of a
turtle was all I found
I frantically looked all through my documents and began to frown.

Then I discovered I was looking at my presentation
through a different view
All was still there, and there was no problem I had to undo.

I went on to admire my daughter's amazing photography
Watching the ocean videos made me feel peaceful and at ease.

I figured out how to expand the videos for a bigger view
Others could enjoy our fabulous adventure, too.

Then I came to the last slide, the one dedicated to you.

The tears began to flow down my cheeks and then they started to pour
It was time to release, but I knew there would be more.

Today was my dad's birthday, too
He passed a few years ago and now both of you

Are floating in the heavens and floating in the clouds
While I am still down here on earth, here on the ground

Working on projects that I hold dear to my heart
Just one way of self-healing, one way to start.

I hope I will be able to present my self-healing artistic piece for all to see
With hopes to bring someone else a method of self-healing
and inner peace.

Personal Reflection

Caritas Touch, so Divine
April 7

Entering a thought made five days ago, validating the
feeling, lovingkindness
experience when I am connected with family and friends.

Energy to heal, energy to feel well
The rejuvenation so mighty that we must tell.

All who are touched, they all will find
That the Caritas touch has been felt and is so divine.

Personal Reflection

This Time I am not Late
April 8

April 8
I just finished listening to my last class and discovered it is not too late

To appreciate a gift I tuck away inside
One that might be disturbing, so I hide

My voice, my singing voice, would you believe
I just listened to a tape of me singing and now I see

That when I am belting out the melody
My voice, my music, the sound, is beautiful to me.

Personal Reflection

Use the Fine China My Dear
April 7

Eid Mubarak up in heaven
Oops! It is not today, it is tomorrow.

A day of happiness and cheer
There will be strong moments of sadness and tears,

For you are not with us to tell us to get up and pray
You are only going to be here in spirit that day.

I hope I can hold it together as the memories of past
celebrations pass through
Pass through my mind as I think of you.

In the beginning I would avoid waking up in the morning on
Eid to go to the Mosque
We would pretend to be sleeping and only go if we must.

I wish I had the days to do over again
We would have been ready to go to prayer and then

Off to the many houses to celebrate
Fasting is over and it is time to fill our bellies and rest after we eat.

I miss you so much and wish you were here
To tell us not to use paper plates and to use the fine china, my dear.

It hurts in my belly, and it hurts in my heart
I know you are no longer suffering, and it is time for me to start

Becoming more independent and less reliant
Time to but on my big girl shoes and show

I can walk the walk to manage my life
Alone without worry and strife.

You taught me how to work through life's events
It's time for me to face them alone.

I do have my family by my side
To ask for a second or third opinion, if they do not mind.

Time to go and start my day
Up early, come what may.

Thank you for being there by my side
I will go forward knowing this with my head held high.

Personal Reflection

Missing in Action
April 10

Missing in action! I was working on my stories, poetry, and the grandkids were over.

Personal Reflection

Eid Mubarak to You in the Heavens Above
April 11

I think I missed writing again, but just to let you know,
life has not been a bore
I am preparing to send out my books and poetry to be published.

I will make you proud, for as my projects come through
Others will be able to cherish my thoughts of honoring you.

Now, check on me from time to time
To see what I've been doing and how I've kept in line.

Today is our second Eid day celebration without you
My challenge today is to welcome the family into a clean house, too.

Remember those days when we'd work together as a team?
You would cook this enormous meal while I cleaned.

Each year we all would have a heated discussion
over china or paper plates
You would always win hands-down that china it was, no mistake.

We will use the china or the new plates today
The paper plates will just have to stay

In the cupboard to come out at a later date
For breakfast, an omelet and toast will be simply great.

Eid Mubarak to you in the heavens above
I miss you greatly, but please be here in spirit, or you will miss all the fun.

Personal Reflection

So Many Things That You Used to Do
April 12

The day has been busy as I try to assemble and arrange my poetry and stories so they will be presentable to the person who will be making them come alive. I hope to have your friend's son create books for me when Zebe goes to Pakistan.

Today was nice. Sophia and the grandkids were here
They watched a movie, relaxed awhile, then packed up their gear.

Off home to rest, busy weekend planned, where we will start out for a lunch at our nephew's house and then
Back home for me so I can dive into my poetry again.

Next week will be busy too, because our palm trees will need to be taken down
I went out a couple of days ago and just the thought of losing them made me frown

They are stately and tall
Another big wind and they may fall

On my house or the neighbor's house—this you knew
It is goodbye to those gorgeous trees that have stood by us so true.

Need to paint the house and power wash it too
Many things you used to organize and do.

Now it is my responsibility; let's see how it goes
Much to learn, so much to know.

Modern technology is moving along
While I sit here with an ancient iPhone.

Time to catch up to the modern world
Just thinking about it makes my mind swirl.

That is enough; now it's time for bed
I'll fluff up my pillow and lay down my head.

Good night, everyone.

Personal Reflection

Late But Not Forgotten
April 13

I guess this entry is going to be late

Late but not forgotten; I just want to say
What a fabulous time I had that day.

Our third Eid spent with family
We had great food.

Personal Reflection

Another Day of First: Taxes
April 14

It is Tax Day tomorrow
Time to reach deep into my pockets with sorrow.

I guess when you do not pay taxes up front
It adds up and you can really be stumped.

If you do not put a nest egg away during the year
The money owed will shock you, I fear.

This will be another one of those firsts for me
Another lesson to go down in my history.

I fear it is not for me
Budgeting the household was your cup of tea.

Personal Reflection

Seven Sutras: Which one Sings to Me
April 15

Seven Sutras; which one sings to me
"Spirit" is my answer.

What are you telling me today
What message do you want to say?

As I join my fellow friends
How can they give me a helping hand

To release the words so poetically versed
Too many to count and never rehearsed.

I am here and open my mind, spirit, and heart
Send me a message even though we're apart.

I am holding it together the best I can
But will always be alert to that open hand.

Personal Reflection

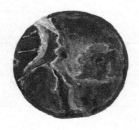

The Image That I See
April 15

The image that I see
Is it me?

I see an elder speaking in my ear
Who has a secret that you hold dear.

Do you have a magical way to display
How you are feeling today?

How do you rid yourself of the sorrow and stress you feel
Do you know a way for me to heal?

You whisper, "Open your heart and mind
That is where the answer is that you seek; and you will find

Ways to detect your inner peace
That is how your stress will be released."

Questions for Reflection

*How are you today? What are the thoughts racing through your mind?
Allow yourself time to reflect on them. Then let them go.*

An Imposing Loss
April 16

Today I said goodbye to a couple more beloved friends
As they waved goodbye with their towering limbs.

I grappled with cutting them
I knew if I did not, someday they would tumble

Fall on my house or a next-door neighbor's
Today was the day I lost a few.

A few more palm trees are now on the ground
The last one took about five strong guys, and a rope tied to a car before
it was down.

The palm tree top plummeted
Impacting the greenery that was around the base of the trees,
taking out other plants.

Tomorrow more trees will be cut down, the last two
I say goodbye, my lofty friends, I will miss you.

Personal Reflection

Closure
April 19

Last entry for *Caregiver's Poetic Journal* but that doesn't mean
I'll stop writing.

Now is the time to wrap up and say
It's time to set down the pen for another day.

Time to rest mind, body, and soul
There will be time to create another, I know.

For now, this chapter is ending, and I open a new door
What will happen I don't know but have much to explore.

As I say a goodbye and close my book
I am also saying goodbye to long-time friends; let's take a look.

The trees which we planted long ago
Are now just a memory, with the seeds once sown.

The family we built grows every day
Before you know it, the little ones will be climbing new trees as they play.

Everyone, everything has a time and place in this world of ours
Sometimes that time feels too short while you shoot for the stars.

I need to remember to slow down the time that's been given to me
Be thankful and grateful.

Just as our lives and families grow and change
So will the garden we created; it will never be the same.

The seedlings will sprout, the trees will bear fruit,
I will continue to cherish the memories of all we have built.

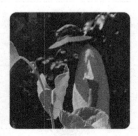

Personal Reflection

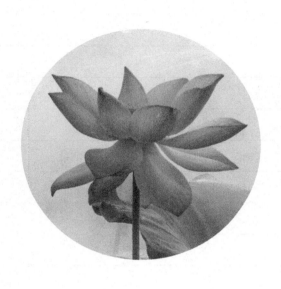

ABOUT THE AUTHOR

Sandra Marie Mohsan, CRN, BSN, PHN, TNP, Caritas Coach®, Charge Nurse

I have been in nursing for forty years. What an amazing journey! So many people have touched my life, and I've had the privilege of touching many lives as well. I have ventured into many specialized fields of nursing and am presently retired as a Kaiser Permanente, Telehealth Advice Charge Nurse, assisting our members throughout Northern California for the last twenty-two years.

In my circle of adventures, I met a nurse who introduced me to Jean Watson's Caring Science, and that is where my artistic appreciation burst into brilliance. Music, dance, poetry, and drawings have poured from me like a fountain of youth. They've rejuvenated me, raised my awareness, and helped me acknowledge many talents. They've made me vibrant and whole. I express my most personal thoughts and emotions through the arts. Now I am ready to start a new journey to show others there is healing in art, and artistic expression brings light into darkness. Artistic expression of our innermost thoughts through the arts helps us maintain a sense of balance and equanimity, renewing us.

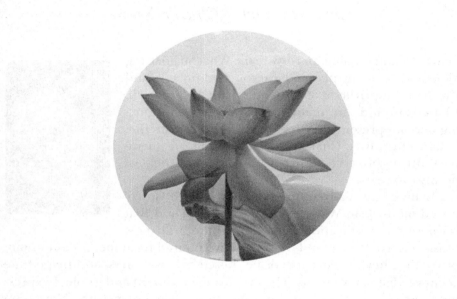

RESOURCES

When you are ready to connect, to take the next step with Sandra, here are more resources to help you in your journey through grief and loss:

Reach Out and Share Your Story

Send your story or an entry from your journal through sandramohsan.com or post in Sandra's Facebook group.

Invite Sandra to Your Workshop

Sandra is available virtually and in person to share her journey through her own grief and loss, how she's working on coping and healing from those losses, and to share practical ways for others to cope and heal from their own grief.

Join a Grief and Loss Group

www.Facebook.com/groups/CopingwithGriefLoss

Join Sandra's Facebook group "Coping with Grief and Loss" for additional support. Experience and create community with others while learning and sharing ways to cope, embrace grief and loss, and find new ways to heal.

Additional Resources

- » The Nursing Way Blog
  www.thenursingway.com/blog
- » Watson's Caring Science Institute
  www.watsoncaringscience.org

Sandra Mohsan

SandraMohsan.com | Sandra@SandraMohsan.com

THANK YOU

Thank you for opening your heart to explore the healing process of journaling. This is my first book and your support is so important. I deeply appreciate you purchasing my book and encourage you to leave a review on Amazon so it will reach more readers. Your thoughts, feedback, and comments will help others understand how this book might help them in their daily lives. My sincere thanks to you in advance for leaving a review.

Made in the USA
Las Vegas, NV
03 December 2024